Table of Contents

PREVIEW

Heart disease is the leading killer of men and women—and claims more lives than all forms of cancer combined. Being diagnosed with cardiovascular disease can also take an emotional toll, affecting your mood, outlook, and quality of life. While weight control and regular exercise are critical for keeping your heart in shape, the food you eat can matter just as much. In fact, along with other healthy lifestyle choices, a heart-healthy diet may reduce your risk of heart disease or stroke by 80%.

No single food can make you magically healthy, so your overall dietary pattern is more important than specific foods. Instead of fried, processed food, packaged meals, and sugary snacks, a heart-healthy diet is built around "real," natural food—fresh from the ground, ocean, or farm.

Whether you're looking to improve your cardiovascular health, have already been diagnosed with heart disease, or have high cholesterol or high blood pressure, these heart-healthy diet tips can help you better manage these conditions and lower your risk of a heart attack.

The first step toward heart health is understanding your risk of heart disease. Your risk depends on many factors, some of which are changeable and others that are not. Risk factors are conditions or habits that make a person more likely to develop a disease.

Heart disease is a leading cause of death in the United States for both men and women. But you can do a lot to protect your heart and stay healthy.

Heart-healthy living involves understanding your risk, making healthy choices, and taking steps to reduce your chances of getting heart disease, including coronary heart disease, the most common type. By taking preventive measures, you can lower your risk of developing heart disease that could lead to a heart attack. You can also improve your overall health and well-being.

HEART HEALTHY DIET RECIPES

BREAKFAST

1. Sausage Egg & Potato Burritos

Prep Time: 15 Minutes

Cook Time: 20 Minutes

Servings: 8

Ingredients

- 1 tablespoon Avocado Oil
- 16 ounces Frozen Diced Hash Brown Potatoes
- 1 cup Bell Pepper any color, chopped
- 1 cup Onion chopped
- ½ cup Fully Cooked Turkey Sausage Crumbles
- 1 teaspoon Salt Free Fiesta Lime Seasoning Blend
- 6 large Eggs whisked
- 4 ounces Reduced Fat Mexican Style Four Cheese Blend
- 2 large Roma Tomatoes about 1 cup chopped
- 8 tortillas Low Carb Flour Tortillas - Taco (42g)
- 1-2 Jalapeno Pepper diced

Instructions

1. Heat oil in a large nonstick skillet over medium heat. Add hash brown potatoes and cook for 5 minutes. Add bell pepper and onion. Cook and stir another 5 minutes, or until potatoes are browned and veggies are soft. Stir in sausage crumbles and seasoning blend.

2. Add eggs to skillet. Cook, stirring occasionally, until eggs are set and fluffy. Remove from heat.
3. Warm tortillas according to package directions and lay out on a flat work surface. Divide egg mixture evenly between the eight tortillas. Sprinkle with cheese, tomatoes and jalapenos. Fold one side of tortilla over mixture and roll to make a burrito. Serve with your favorite hot sauce. Makes 8 burritos

To Make Ahead:

1. Let completed burritos cool. Wrap individually in plastic wrap and place inside a food storage bag. Refrigerate for up to 3 days. Freeze for up to 2 months
2. To Reheat: Unwrap burrito and rewrap with a paper towel. Microwave 1-3 minutes at 50% power. Add a minute or two more if from frozen.

2. Tater Tot Casserole
Prep Time: 20 Minutes

Cook Time: 1hr 2 Minutes

Servings: 12

Ingredients

- 1 pound Ground Turkey Sausage
- ½ cup Onion chopped
- 12 large Eggs
- ½ cup 2% Milk
- ¼ teaspoon Kosher Salt
- ¼ teaspoon Black Pepper
- 1 (32-ounce) bag Frozen Tater Tots
- 4 ounces Reduced Fat Monterey Jack Cheese shredded
- 6 ounces Reduced Fat Cheddar Cheese shredded
- ¼ cup Green Onions sliced

Instructions

1. Preheat oven to 350°F. Coat a 9x13-inch baking dish with cooking spray.
2. Cook the sausage and onion in a large nonstick skillet over medium-high heat for 5 minutes, or until sausage is no longer pink and onions are soft. Drain on a paper towel lined plate.
3. Whisk together eggs, milk, salt, and pepper in a large bowl. Stir in Monterey jack cheese and 1 cup cheddar cheese.

4. Arrange tater tots in a single layer in prepared baking dish. Evenly top with drained sausage and onion mixture. Pour egg mixture over it all.
5. Bake in preheated oven for 40-45 minutes, or until eggs are set. Sprinkle with remaining cheddar cheese and bake another 5 minutes, or until cheese is melted.
6. Let casserole sit for 10 minutes before cutting into 12 servings. Garnish with green onions.

3. Freezer Sandwiches
Prep Time: 5 Minutes

Cook Time: 15 Minutes

Servings: 12

Ingredients

- 12 large Eggs
- ⅔ cup 2% Milk
- ¼ teaspoon Kosher Salt
- ¼ teaspoon Black Pepper
- 12 Whole Wheat English Muffin split
- Butter Flavor Cooking Spray
- 12 slices Reduced Fat Cheddar Cheese
- 12 slices Canadian Bacon

Instructions

1. Preheat oven to 325°F. Lightly coat a 13x9-inch baking pan with cooking spray and set aside.

Cook the Eggs:

2. In a large bowl, whisk together eggs, milk, salt, and pepper. Pour into prepared baking dish. Bake in preheated oven for 15-18 minutes, or until set. Remove from oven and cool on a wire rack. Cut cooled eggs into 12 square portions.

Assemble the Sandwiches:

3. While eggs are cooking in the oven, toast the English Muffins. Lightly coat toasted muffins with cooking spray, if desired.
4. Layer each sandwich in the following order-
5. Muffin Bottom, Egg Portion, Cheese Slice, Canadian Bacon, Muffin Top
6. Wrap each sandwich in plastic wrap. Place six wrapped sandwiches inside each labeled 1-gallon freezer bag.

To Reheat in Microwave:

1. Remove plastic wrap from frozen sandwich and wrap sandwich in a paper towel. Microwave for 1-3 minutes total cooking time, flipping sandwich over halfway through. Every microwave is different, so test what works best. For me, I microwave for 90 seconds at 70% power, flip the sandwich and microwave for another 90 seconds at 70% power.

4. Low Cholesterol Sausage Wraps

Prep Time: 15 Minutes

Cook Time: 10 Minutes

Servings: 4

Ingredients

- 1 tablespoon Grapeseed Oil
- 1 cup Fully Cooked Turkey Sausage Crumbles
- 1 cup Mushrooms chopped
- ½ cup Green Bell Pepper chopped
- ¼ teaspoon Salt Free Chili Powder
- ⅛ teaspoon Kosher Salt
- ¼ teaspoon Black Pepper
- 1 cup Liquid Egg Substitute
- 4 Low Carb Flour Tortillas soft taco (42g each)
- 1 Tomato chopped

Instructions

Cook the Veggies and Eggs

2. Heat oil in a large nonstick skillet over medium heat. Add mushrooms, bell pepper, chili powder, salt and pepper. Cook and stir 3 minutes or until vegetables are tender. Stir in the sausage crumbles.
3. Pour in egg substitute. Let egg mixture set around edge of skillet. Run a spatula around set edges, lifting mixture so uncooked portion can flow underneath. Continue process until egg is cooked through. Remove from heat. Cover to keep warm until ready to assemble wraps.

Assemble and Serve

1. Microwave tortillas on high for 30 seconds. Divide mixture evenly between 4 tortillas and top with chopped tomato. Wrap "burrito" style. Serve with hot sauce if desired.
2. Make-Ahead Instructions
3. Cook the Veggies and Eggs as directed above. Let mixture cool. Store in airtight container in fridge for up to 5 days.

5. Low Sodium Chimichurri Tostadas
Prep Time: 20 Minutes

Cook Time: 10 Minutes

Servings: 4

Ingredients

- ½ cup Fresh Parsley
- ¼ cup Fresh Oregano
- 2 tablespoons Red Wine Vinegar
- 2 cloves Garlic cut in half
- ½ teaspoon Ground Cumin
- ½ teaspoon Salt Free Chili Powder
- ¼ teaspoon Kosher Salt
- ⅛ teaspoon Black Pepper
- ⅓ cup Avocado Oil
- ½ teaspoon Crushed Red Pepper
- 1 (15-ounce) can No Salt Added Black Beans drained and rinsed

Avocado Oil Spray

- 4 large Eggs
- 4 Tostada Shells Ortega shells don't have any Saturated Fat
- ¼ cup Queso Fresco or Cotija Cheese crumbled

Instructions

Make the Chimichurri

1. Place the first 8 ingredients in a food processor. Add avocado oil and optional crushed red pepper. Pulse until desired consistency. Cover and refrigerate until ready to serve.
2. Warm the Beans and Cook the Eggs
3. Warm the beans in a saucepan over medium heat.
4. Meanwhile, heat buttery spread and avocado oil in a nonstick skillet over medium-high heat. Break eggs into pan, 1 at a time; Reduce heat to low. Cook until whites are set and yolks cooked as desired.

Plate and Serve

1. Microwave tostada shells according to box directions.
2. Divide warmed beans evenly between shells. Top with equal amounts of cheese. Add fried egg and chimichurri sauce.

6. Ham & Cheese Potatoes
Prep Time: 10 Minutes

Cook Time: 30 Minutes

Servings: 8

Ingredients

- 1 (28-ounce) package Frozen O'Brien Potatoes with Onion and Peppers
- 1 pound Ham Steak diced into bite-size pieces
- 1 (10.75-ounce) can Cream of Celery Soup
- ½ teaspoon Black Pepper
- ¼ cup Parmesan Cheese shredded
- 1 cup Reduced Fat Sharp Cheddar Cheese shredded

Instructions

Make the Casserole

1. Preheat oven to 400°F. Lightly spray 13 x 9 inch baking dish with cooking spray. Set aside.
2. In a large mixing bowl, combine potatoes, ham, soup, and pepper. Pour mixture into prepared baking dish. Bake, uncovered for 25 minutes. Top with cheeses and cook another 5-10 minutes or until cheese is melted. Remove from oven and cool for at least 10 minutes.

7. Simple Cheese and Mushroom Omelets

Prep Time: 5 Minutes

Cook Time: 10 Minutes

Servings: 4

Ingredients

- 3 tablespoon Avocado Oil
- 8 ounces Mushrooms sliced
- 6 large Eggs
- ½ cup Liquid Egg Whites
- ¼ cup 2% Milk
- ¼ teaspoon Kosher Salt
- ¼ teaspoon Black Pepper
- 2 ounces Reduced Fat Monterey Jack Cheese shredded

Instructions

1. In a 4-cup glass measuring cup, whisk eggs, egg whites, milk, salt, and pepper. There should be 2 cups total mixture.
2. In a nonstick skillet, heat oil over medium-high heat. Add the mushrooms and sauté for 3-5 minutes, or until soft. Transfer mushrooms to a bowl. Wipe skillet.
3. Add ½ tablespoon oil to the skillet and heat over medium. Add ½ cup of the egg mixture and rotate pan to ensure even layer. Cook for 2 minutes, lifting edges slightly to let uncooked egg flow under cooked portion. Add 2 tablespoons cheese and about ¼ cup

of the mushrooms to one side of eggs. Fold over into an omelet with a spatula. Transfer omelet to a plate. Cover to keep warm until ready to serve. Repeat process to complete 3 more omelets.

Make Ahead:

1. Cooked and cooled omelets can be refrigerated up to 5 days. Package individually as a meal, or, layer several omelets in one container with waxed paper in between. Reheat in the microwave.

8. Buttermilk Pancakes
Prep Time: 5 Minutes

Cook Time: 5 Minutes

Servings: 4

Ingredients

- 1 large Egg
- 2 tablespoons Canola Oil
- 1 cup Water
- 1½ cups Heart Healthy Buttermilk Pancake Mix
- 2 tablespoons Buttery Spread
- 1 cup Sugar Free Pancake Syrup

Instructions

2. Preheat griddle and coat with cooking spray.
3. Combine egg, oil, and water in a medium bowl. Whisk in pancake mix until well blended. Let stand for 5 minutes.
4. Pour batter onto hot griddle in 5-inch circles. Cook until edges look dry and middle has bubbles. Turn over with a spatula and cook for another minute, or until bottoms are golden brown.
5. Recipe makes 8 (5-inch) pancakes.
6. Each serving = 2 pancakes, ½ tablespoon buttery spread, and ¼ cup of syrup.

9. Skillet Frittata Florentine

Prep Time: 15 Minutes

Cook Time: 15 Minutes

Servings: 4

Ingredients

- 1½ tablespoons Grapeseed Oil
- 6 large Eggs
- ½ teaspoon Dried Basil Leaves
- ½ teaspoon Dried Oregano
- ¼ teaspoon Garlic Powder
- ¼ teaspoon Kosher Salt
- ¼ teaspoon Black Pepper
- ½ cup Onion chopped
- ½ cup Red Bell Pepper chopped
- 1 cup Baby Spinach
- 2 tablespoons Real Bacon Bits
- 2 ounces Reduced Fat Mozzarella Cheese shredded

Instructions

1. Preheat oven to 350°F.
2. Whisk eggs, basil, oregano, garlic powder, salt, and pepper in a small bowl and set aside.
3. Heat oil in an 8-inch nonstick, ovenproof skillet over medium-high heat. Add onion and bell pepper. Cook and stir 5 minutes, or until tender. Reduce heat to medium-low and add spinach.
4. Pour in egg mixture and bacon bits. As eggs set, push cooked portions toward the center to let uncooked

eggs flow underneath. Cook until eggs are almost set. Remove from heat and sprinkle with cheese.

5. Bake in preheated oven for 10 minutes, or until eggs are set and cheese is melted. Remove from oven and let cool 5 minutes. Cut in four wedges.

10. Roast Beef Pinwheels
Prep Time: 10 Minutes

Cook Time: 15 Minutes

Servings: 8

Ingredients

- 1 (8-ounce) tube Refrigerated Crescent Dough Sheet such as Pillsbury
- 2 tablespoons Dijon Mustard
- 8 slices Reduced Fat Provolone Cheese
- 8 ounces Low Sodium Roast Beef sliced thin
- ½ cup Red Bell Pepper chopped

Instructions

1. Preheat oven to 375°F. Line a baking sheet with parchment paper and set aside.
2. Unroll crescent dough and cut in half lengthwise. Spread each rectangle with 1 tablespoon of mustard. Top each rectangle with half the cheese slices and roast beef. Overlap if needed to fit on dough. Sprinkle bell pepper on top.
3. Roll up each rectangle, jelly-roll style, starting with the short side. Pinch seams to seal. Cut each roll crosswise into 4 slices. Place on prepared baking sheet, cut side down. Bake in preheated oven for 15 minutes, or until golden brown.

LUNCH

11. Hot Brown Party Rolls
Prep Time: 20 Minutes

Cook Time: 25 Minutes

Servings: 12

Ingredients

- 1 (12-count) package Sweet Hawaiian Slider Buns such as Pepperidge Farm
- 6 slice Ultra Thin Swiss Cheese
- 8 ounces Low Sodium Deli Turkey
- 1 Tomato sliced thin
- 6 slices Thick Cut Bacon cooked and cut in 2-inch pieces
- 1 ounce Parmesan Cheese shredded
- ½ cup Buttery Spread melted
- 1 tablespoon Dijon Mustard
- 2 teaspoons Dried Minced Onion
- 1½ teaspoons Worcestershire Sauce
- 1 teaspoon Light Brown Sugar
- ½ teaspoon Dried Minced Garlic
- ½ teaspoon Hot Sauce such as Cholula
- Avocado Oil Spray

Instructions

1. Preheat oven to 375°F. Lightly spray 11x7-inch baking dish with avocado oil.
2. Split rolls, without separating individually. Place bottom rolls in prepared baking dish.

Build the sandwich layers:

1. Fold 3 slices of cheese into quarters. Lay one section of cheese on each roll bottom in baking dish. Add turkey slices, folding to fit in an even layer. Place tomato slices in even layer. Top with bacon pieces. Fold remaining 3 slices of cheese into quarters and top each roll with cheese section. Sprinkle evenly with Parmesan cheese. Cover with top roll halves.

Bake the Rolls:

2. In a 2-cup liquid measuring cup, stir together the melted butter, Dijon mustard, minced onion, Worcestershire sauce, brown sugar, minced garlic, and the hot sauce. Slowly pour mixture over the rolls, allowing mixture to soak into rolls. Cover dish with foil and bake in preheated oven for 15 minutes. Remove foil and bake another 5-10 minutes, or until tops of rolls are lightly browned. Remove from oven and let stand 5 minutes before serving.

12. Garden Scrambled Eggs
Prep Time: 20 Minutes

Cook Time: 5 Minutes

Servings: 4

Ingredients

- ⅓ cup Roma Tomatoes chopped
- ⅓ cup Onion chopped
- ⅓ cup Bell Peppers chopped
- 4 large Eggs
- ½ cup Liquid Egg Whites pick good quality 100% egg whites
- 2 tablespoons Fresh Parsley chopped
- 6 tablespoons Light Sour Cream
- 1 tablespoon Dijon Mustard
- ⅛ teaspoon Kosher Salt
- ⅛ teaspoon Black Pepper
- Avocado Oil Cooking Spray

Instructions

3. Spray a large nonstick skillet with cooking spray. Heat pan over medium heat. Add veggies and coat with cooking spray. Cook and stir for 3 minutes, or until veggies are tender.
4. While veggies are cooking, whisk together eggs, egg whites, parsley, sour cream, Dijon, salt, and pepper.
5. Add egg mixture to skillet. Heat over medium for 2 minutes. Let eggs begin to set around edges and bottom. Run a heat-resistant spatula around edges

and through pan to form large curds. Continue cooking until eggs are set.

6. Divide evenly between four plates and serve.

13. Hash Brown Frittata
Prep Time: 10 Minutes

Cook Time: 25 Minutes

Servings: 6

Ingredients

- 6 large Eggs
- ½ cup Half and Half
- ½ teaspoon Black Pepper
- ¾ teaspoon Kosher Salt divided
- 3 tablespoons Canola Oil
- ½ cup Onion chopped
- 1 (20-ounce) package Refrigerated Shredded Hash Browns such as Simply Potatoes
- 1 teaspoon Dried Dill Weed

Instructions

1. Preheat oven to 375°F.
2. In a medium bowl, whisk together, eggs, half-and-half, dried dill weed, ½ teaspoon salt, and pepper.
3. Heat 1 tablespoon oil in a large (10-12-inches) nonstick, oven safe skillet over medium high heat. Add onion. Cook and stir as needed for 5 minutes, or until onion is softened. Add 1 tablespoon of oil and rotate skillet to coat bottom of pan. Add hash browns and spread out in an even layer. Cook for 5-6 minutes, or until browned on bottom. With a wide spatula, flip hash browns in sections, trying to rotate top to bottom. Sprinkle remaining ¼ teaspoon salt and 1

tablespoon oil over top of hash browns. Cook for 3-4 minutes, or until bottoms are browned.

4. Reduce heat to medium. Pour egg mixture over hash browns in skillet. Cook, undisturbed, for 2-3 minutes, or until outer edges are set. Transfer skillet to preheated oven and bake for 6-8 minutes. Frittata is done when middle of eggs are set. Remove from oven. Loosen edges with a spatula and turn frittata out onto a cutting board. Let sit for 5 minutes.
5. Cut into six wedges and garnish with pico de gallo, if desired.

14. Huevos Rancheros
Prep Time: 30 Minutes

Cook Time: 30 Minutes

Servings: 8

Ingredients

Sauce:

- 4 Roma Tomatoes rough chop
- 3 cloves Garlic
- 1 pepper Chipotle Peppers in Adobo Sauce add some of the sauce for more heat
- ½ cup Onion chopped
- 1 teaspoon Ground Cumin
- ½ teaspoon Kosher Salt
- 1 tablespoon Avocado Oil
- ¼ cup Cilantro chopped
- ½ Lime

Beans:

- 3 tablespoons Avocado Oil
- ½ cup Onion chopped
- 3 cloves Garlic chopped fine
- 1 teaspoon Ground Cumin
- 2 (15-ounce) cans Low Sodium Pinto Beans drained and rinsed
- ½ teaspoon Kosher Salt
- ½ Lime

Assembly:

- 8 large Eggs
- 8 (42g-47g) Flour or Corn Tortillas
- 4 tablespoons Queso Fresca Cheese
- 1 Jalapeno Pepper seeded and sliced

Instructions

Make the Sauce:

1. In a Food Processor or a Blender, puree the tomatoes, garlic, chipotle pepper, onion, cumin, salt, and ¼ cup water.
2. Heat 1 tablespoon avocado oil in a medium saucepan over medium heat. Add the tomato puree and bring to a simmer. Cook and stir for about 6 minutes, or until sauce is slightly thickened. Stir in Cilantro and juice from ½ a lime. Keep warm until ready to serve.

Cook the Beans:

1. Heat 3 tablespoons avocado oil in a large skillet over medium heat. Add onion and cook for 7-8 minutes, until onion is soft. Stir in garlic and cumin. Add the beans, salt, and 1 cup water. Cook, mashing the beans with a potato masher, for 5-6 minutes, or until the beans are thick and still chunky. Stir in juice from ½ lime. Keep warm until ready to serve.

Assemble and Serve:

2. Coat large nonstick skillet with Avocado Spray. Heat skillet over medium heat. Add the eggs and lightly Salt and Pepper. Cover and cook until whites of eggs are set, about 3-4 minutes.
3. Warm tortillas according to package directions.

4. Top each tortilla with beans, fried egg, sauce, cheese, jalapeno slices, and cilantro.

15. Egg and Tomato Scramble
Prep Time: 30 Minutes

Cook Time: 30 Minutes

Servings: 8

Ingredients

- 2 Roma Tomatoes chopped
- 2 teaspoons Dried Basil Leaves
- 4 large Eggs
- 1 cup Liquid Egg Whites
- ½ teaspoon Minced Garlic (jar)
- 2 teaspoons Grapeseed Oil
- ¼ teaspoon Kosher Salt
- ¼ teaspoon Black Pepper

Instructions

1. Combine tomato and basil in a small bowl and set aside.
2. In another bowl, beat eggs, liquid egg whites, garlic, salt and pepper. Heat oil in a large nonstick skillet. Add egg mixture and cook until egg is almost set. Add tomato mixture. Cook and stir until egg is completely set.
3. Divide scrambled eggs evenly between 4 plates and serve.

16. Banana Chocolate Chip Muffin
Prep Time: 10 Minutes

Cook Time: 25 Minutes

Servings: 12

Ingredients

- 3 ripe Bananas peeled and mashed with a fork
- 2 large Eggs
- 6 tablespoons Light Brown Sugar
- ½ cup Light Sour Cream
- 3 tablespoons Canola Oil
- 1⅓ cups All Purpose Flour
- 1½ teaspoons Baking Powder
- ½ teaspoon Baking Soda
- ¾ teaspoon Ground Cinnamon
- ⅛ teaspoon Table Salt
- 3 tablespoons Mini Chocolate Chips

Instructions

1. Preheat oven to 350°F. Lightly spray with cooking oil 12-cup muffin pan, or line with paper cups.
2. In a medium bowl, whisk eggs, sugar, sour cream, and oil until smooth.
3. In a large bowl, mix flour, baking powder, baking soda, cinnamon, and salt. Make a well in the center of flour mixture and mix in the egg mixture, Combine well, but not overbeat. Fold in the bananas and chocolate chips.

4. Fill each prepared muffin cup about three-quarters full with the batter. Bake the muffins in preheated oven for 20-25 minutes, or until set.
5. Remove muffins from oven and let sit in pan for 5 minutes. Transfer to a wire rack to cool completely.
6. Makes 12 muffins.

17. Reduced Fat Sausage Gravy and Biscuits
Prep Time: 5 Minutes

Cook Time: 20 Minutes

Servings: 10

Ingredients

- 1 pound Reduced Fat Pork Sausage
- ⅓ cup All Purpose Flour
- 3-4 cups 2% Milk
- ½ teaspoon Salt Free Seasoning Salt
- 1 teaspoon Black Pepper
- 2 (6-ounce) tubes Refrigerated Biscuits regular size

Instructions

Make the Sausage Gravy:

1. Break the sausage up with your fingers in a large nonstick skillet. Cook over medium-high heat until no longer pink. Reduce heat to medium-low and sprinkle half the flour on top. Cook and stir for 1 minute. Repeat with last half of flour.
2. Pour in the milk. Cook and stir constantly until gravy thickens, about 10-12 minutes. Stir in the seasoned salt and pepper. Keep gravy on lowest heat setting until ready to serve. Stir as needed.

Bake the Biscuits:

1. Bake the biscuits according to package directions. Remove from oven and keep warm until ready to serve.

Plate and Serve:

2. Each serving is one biscuit and about ⅓ cup of gravy.
3. Refrigerate any leftover gravy in an airtight container for up to 3 days.

18. Spinach and Ham Quiche

Prep Time: 20 Minutes

Cook Time: 45 Minutes

Servings: 6

Ingredients

- 1 Frozen 9-inch Deep Dish Pie Crust
- 2 tablespoons Avocado Oil
- 1 cup Frozen Chopped Spinach thawed and drained
- ½ cup Onion chopped
- ½ teaspoon Minced Garlic (jar)
- ¼ teaspoon Kosher Salt
- ¼ teaspoon Black Pepper
- 4 ounces Swiss Cheese shredded
- 4 ounces Ham Steak cubed
- 6 large Eggs
- 1 cup 2% Milk

Instructions

1. Preheat oven to 375°F.
2. Heat oil in a large skillet over medium-high heat. Add spinach and onion. Cook and stir 5-7 minutes, or until onion is tender. Add garlic and cook 1 minute. Stir in salt and pepper. Spoon into pie crust. Top with ham and cheese.
3. Whisk eggs and milk in a bowl until blended. Pour over mixture in pie crust.
4. Bake on lower rack of preheated oven for 35-40 minutes, or until set. Check crust about half way

through baking and wrap with foil if browning too
quickly.

5. Let rest 10 minutes before cutting into 6 equal slices.

19. Chicken Cordon Blue Quiche
Prep Time: 20 Minutes

Cook Time: 30 Minutes

Servings: 6

Ingredients

- 2 teaspoons Dijon Mustard
- 1 Frozen 9-inch Deep Dish Pie Crust
- 1 cup Cooked Chicken shredded or cubed
- 3 ounces Black Forest Ham chopped
- 2 tablespoons Green Onions chopped
- 2 ounces Swiss Cheese shredded
- 1 cup 2% Milk
- 4 large Eggs
- ⅛ teaspoon Kosher Salt
- ⅛ teaspoon Black Pepper

Instructions

1. Place a rimmed baking sheet in the middle of the oven and preheat to 425°F.
2. Spread the mustard on the bottom of the pie crust. Layer with the chicken, ham, green onions, and cheese.
3. Whisk together the eggs, milk, salt, and pepper. Pour over the filling in the pie crust.
4. Carefully set the pie pan on the hot baking sheet. Bake 30 minutes, or until the eggs are set.
5. Let quiche rest for 5 minutes before cutting.

20. Mexican Skillet Dinner with Homemade Chorizo

Prep Time: 20 Minutes

Cook Time: 15 Minutes

Servings: 6

Ingredients

- 1 pound Homemade Chorizo Recipe see below
- 2 cups Frozen Corn
- 1 (14.5-ounce) can No Salt Added Diced Tomatoes undrained
- 1 cup Instant Rice uncooked
- ½ cup Water
- 1 (15-ounce) can Low Sodium Pinto Beans rinsed and drained
- 3 ounces Reduced Fat Mexican Style Four Cheese Blend
- ½ head Iceberg Lettuce shredded for garnish
- 1 Tomato chopped for garnish

Homemade Chorizo:

- 1 pound Ground Pork
- 3 tablespoons Paprika
- ½ tablespoon Ground Cumin
- 1 tablespoon Ancho Chili Powder
- 1 tablespoon Salt Free Chili Powder
- 1 teaspoon Dried Oregano
- 1 teaspoon Ground Coriander
- ½ teaspoon Kosher Salt
- 2 tablespoons White Vinegar
- 1 teaspoon Minced Garlic (jar)

Instructions

1. In a large skillet cook the chorizo over medium heat for 5-7 minutes. Remove chorizo and drain on paper towels. Drain fat from skillet.
2. Mexican Skillet Dinner with Homemade Chorizo plated with a corn tostada
3. In same skillet combine corn, tomatoes with juice, rice, and water. Bring to a boil. Reduce heat and simmer for 5 minutes or until the liquid is absorbed and rice is tender. Stir in the beans and chorizo. Heat through, stirring as needed. Remove from heat. Sprinkle with cheese and cover until cheese has melted.
4. Serve as is or make into tacos, burritos, or like we did here, as a tostada topping.

Homemade Chorizo Recipe:

1. In a small bowl, mix together the paprika, ground cumin, ancho chili powder, chili powder, oregano, coriander, and salt.
2. Homemade Chorizo raw and ready to be cooked
3. In a large bowl, add ground pork, spice mix, vinegar, and garlic. Mix with your hands until well combined.
4. Ready to use in your favorite recipe or store in an airtight container. Freeze for up to 3 months, or refrigerate for up to 3 days.

DINNER
21. Italian Steak Sandwiches
Prep Time: 20 Minutes

Cook Time: 10 Minutes

Servings: 6

Ingredients

- 2 tablespoon High Heat Olive Oil
- 1½ cups Onion sliced thin
- 1½ teaspoons Chopped Garlic (jar)
- ⅛ teaspoon Black Pepper
- 1½ pounds Thin Sliced Beef Sirloin Steak the thinner the better
- ½ cup Fresh Parsley chopped
- 2 ounces Giardiniera rough chop
- 6 (84-grams) each Ciabatta Rolls (84g) split
- 6 slices Reduced Fat Provolone Cheese

Instructions

1. Heat the olive oil in a large nonstick skillet over medium-high heat. Add the steak in batches and cook until browned, about 30 seconds to 1 minute per side. Transfer meat to a bowl and cover to keep warm.
2. In same skillet add onion. Cook and stir as needed 4 minutes. Add garlic and cook for 30 seconds. Add onion and garlic along with any pan juices to the bowl with the steak. Add parsley and toss to coat.

3. Divide the steak and onion mixture evenly between
    the six ciabatta roll bottoms. Top each with
    giardiniera and slice of cheese, the roll top.

22. Lighter King Ranch Chicken Casserole

Prep Time: 20 Minutes

Cook Time: 45 Minutes

Servings: 8

Ingredients

1. 1 cup Hot Water
2. 1 teaspoon Sodium Free Chicken Bouillon Granules such as Herb-Ox
3. 1 tablespoon Canola Oil
4. 1 cup Onion chopped
5. 1 cup Red Bell Pepper chopped
6. 1 cup Green Bell Pepper chopped
7. 1 (10.5-ounce) can Less Sodium Cream of Mushroom Soup such as Healthy Request
8. 1 (10.5-ounce) can Less Sodium Cream of Chicken Soup such as Healthy Request
9. 1 (10-ounce) can No Salt Added Diced Tomatoes with Green Chilies
10. 2 tablespoon Light Sour Cream
11. 2 teaspoons Ground Cumin
12. 1 teaspoon Ancho Chili Powder
13. 1½ teaspoons Chipotle Chili Powder
14. ½ teaspoon Dried Oregano
15. ½ teaspoon Kosher Salt
16. 3 cups Cooked Chicken shredded
17. 8 ounces Reduced Fat Cheddar Cheese shredded
18. 10 (6-inch) Corn Tortillas torn in quarters
19. 2 Jalapeno Pepper sliced

Instructions

1. Preheat oven to 350°F.
2. Stir chicken bouillon granules into hot water until dissolved and set aside.
3. Heat oil in a large nonstick skillet over medium-high heat. Add onion and peppers. Sauté for about 5 minutes, or until veggies are softened. Transfer to a large bowl.
4. Stir in soups, tomatoes with chilies, chicken broth, sour cream, cumin, ancho and chipotle chili powders, oregano, and salt. Combine well.
5. Spread about a ¼ cup of soup mixture in the bottom of a 13 x 9-inch baking dish. Layer with half the chicken, half the soup mixture, half the cheese and half the tortillas.
6. Top tortillas with remaining chicken, half the remaining soup mixture, half of the remaining cheese, and the remaining tortillas. Spread remaining soup mixture over tortillas and top with remaining cheese.
7. Bake uncovered in preheated oven for 40 minutes, or until bubbling. Remove from oven and let rest at least 10 minutes.
8. Divide dish into eight servings and garnish with sliced jalapenos.

23. Arugula & Potato Salad with Fresh Herbs
Prep Time: 20 Minutes

Cook Time: 15 Minutes

Servings: 6

Ingredients

- 1½ pounds Baby Yukon Gold Potatoes cut in half
- ¼ cup Mayonnaise
- ¼ cup Fat Free Plain Greek Yogurt
- 2 tablespoons Lemon Juice
- 1 tablespoon Capers rinsed
- 2 tablespoons Fresh Chives chopped
- 1 tablespoon Fresh Dill chopped
- 1 tablespoon Fresh Parsley chopped
- ¼ teaspoon Kosher Salt
- ¼ teaspoon Black Pepper
- 2½ ounces Baby Arugula

Instructions

Cook the Potatoes:

1. Place potatoes in a large saucepan. Pour enough water in pan to cover potatoes. Bring to a boil. Reduce heat, cover and cook for 10 minutes, or until potatoes are tender, but still firm. Drain and spread potatoes on a baking sheet in a single layer. Cool at least 30 minutes.

Make the Dressing:

2. In a large bowl, whisk the mayonnaise, yogurt, lemon
    juice, mustard, capers, chives, dill, parsley, salt and
    pepper.

Finish the Dish:

3. Add cooled potatoes and arugula to dressing and toss
    to coat. Garnish with fresh herbs as desired.

24. Cheddar Potato Chowder
Prep Time: 25 Minutes

Cook Time: 15 Minutes

Servings: 6

Ingredients

- 2 cups Water
- 5 ounces Red Potatoes cut into bite-size cubes
- 1 cup Carrot sliced
- 1 cup Celery sliced
- ¼ cup Onion chopped
- ¼ teaspoon Kosher Salt
- ¼ teaspoon Black Pepper
- ¼ cup All Purpose Flour
- 2 cups 2% Milk
- 6 ounces Reduced Fat Cheddar Cheese shredded
- 8 ounces Ham Steak cut into bite-size cubes

Instructions

4. In a Dutch oven, stir together water, potatoes, carrots, celery, onion, salt, and pepper. Bring to a boil. Reduce heat, cover, and simmer for 15 minutes, or until veggies are tender.
5. Meanwhile, place flour in a large saucepan and whisk in the milk. Bring to a boil over medium heat. Cook and stir for 2 minutes, or until slightly thickened. Remove from heat and stir in cheese until melted.

6. Stir cheese sauce and ham into Dutch oven with veggies. Heat over low for a couple minutes, or until heated through.
7. Divide chowder evenly between 6 bowls and serve. Leftover servings can be refrigerated up to 3 days and reheated in the microwave.

25. Pan Fried Shrimp with Homemade Cocktail Sauce
Prep Time: 15 Minutes

Cook Time: 5 Minutes

Servings: 6

Ingredients

- 2 cups Plain Panko Crumbs
- 4 tablespoons Cilantro chopped
- 2 pounds Extra Jumbo Shrimp (16-20 per pound) thawed, peeled and deveined
- ½ teaspoon Black Pepper
- 1 large Egg
- 2 teaspoon Water
- 4 tablespoons Canola Oil

Cocktail Sauce:

- 1 cup 50/50 Ketchup (Low Sodium/Low Sugar)
- 2 tablespoons Lemon Juice
- 2 tablespoons Worcestershire Sauce
- 3 tablespoons Prepared Horseradish

Instructions

Prepare the Cocktail Sauce:

1. Combine the ketchup, lemon juice, Worcestershire sauce, and horseradish in a bowl. Cover and refrigerate until ready to serve.

Cook the Shrimp:

2. Place panko and cilantro in a food processor and pulse
   2-3 times, or until mixture is finely minced. Transfer
   to a shallow dish.
3. In another shallow dish, whisk egg and water
   together.
4. Sprinkle shrimp with pepper. In 3 or 4 batches,
   dredge shrimp in egg mixture, then crumb mixture.
   Place on a plate in a single layer. Repeat till all shrimp
   are coated.
5. Heat a large or extra large nonstick skillet over
   medium-high heat. Add 2 tablespoons oil and tilt pan
   to coat. Add half the shrimp in a single layer and cook
   for 2-3 minutes per side, or until golden brown. Drain
   shrimp on a paper towel. Add remaining 2
   tablespoons oil and repeat to cook all the shrimp.

Plate and Serve:

1. Divide shrimp evenly between six plates. Garnish with
   cilantro and serve with about ¼ cup cocktail sauce
   per serving.

26. Everything Spiced Shrimp, Broccoli, and Potatoes
Prep Time: 20 Minutes

Cook Time: 20 Minutes

Servings: 4

Ingredients

- 1½ pounds Baby Red Potatoes cut in quarters
- 1 head Broccoli Crowns cut florets bite-size
- 6 ounces Less Fat Cream Cheese Tub
- ½ teaspoon Freeze Dried Chives
- ½ teaspoon Dried Minced Onion
- 1¼ pounds Large Shrimp peeled and deveined
- 1 tablespoon High Heat Olive Oil
- 1 tablespoon Salt Free Everything Bagel Seasoning
- 1 tablespoon Buttery Spread
- 2 tablespoons Green Onions sliced

Instructions

2. Put potatoes in a large pot and cover with 1 or 2 inches of water. Bring to a boil, then reduce heat. Simmer 12-15 minutes or until potatoes are tender. Add the broccoli and cook 1-2 more minutes, or until broccoli is bright green and crisp-tender. Reserve 3 tablespoons of cooking water, then drain the potatoes and broccoli.
3. Stir cream cheese, dried chives, minced onion, and reserved cooking water in a large bowl until smooth. Add potatoes and broccoli. Stir to coat. Cover to keep warm until ready to serve.

4. Toss the shrimp with oil and everything seasoning in a
    bowl. Heat a large nonstick skillet over medium-high
    heat 2-3 minutes, or until very hot. Add the butter and
    swirl to coat pan. Add the shrimp in a single layer and
    cook 3-4 minutes, or until browned, turning halfway
    through.

27. Skillet Beef, Corn & Zucchini Tater Tot Casserole

Prep Time: 20 Minutes

Cook Time: 30 Minutes

Servings: 6

Ingredients

- 1 pound 93% Lean Ground Beef
- 1 cup Onion chopped
- 2 medium Zucchini sliced, then quartered
- 3 medium Roma Tomatoes chopped
- 1 cup Frozen Corn
- 1 tablespoon Salt Free Chili Powder
- 1 tablespoon Worcestershire Sauce
- ¼ teaspoon Kosher Salt
- 1 tablespoon All Purpose Flour
- 4 ounces Reduced Fat Cheddar Cheese shredded
- 10 ounces Frozen Tater Tots

Instructions

1. Preheat oven to 400°F.
2. Heat an extra large, ovenproof skillet over medium-high heat. Add ground beef and onions. Cook and break up beef with a wooden spoon for 5 minutes, or until the beef is no longer pink. Add zucchini, 1 cup of the tomatoes, corn, chili powder, Worcestershire sauce, and salt. Cook and stir 3-4 minutes. Sprinkle with the flour. Cook and stir 1 minute. Remove from heat.

3. Spread meat and veggie mixture into an even layer. Top with ½ cup of cheese. Arrange tater tots on top in a single layer.
4. Bake in preheated oven for 15 minutes. Sprinkle the remaining cheese on top of tots. Bake another 5 minutes, or until cheese is melted and tots are browned. Remove from oven and garnish with remaining tomatoes.

28. Maple Brined Roast Pork Loin with Mustard Glaze
Prep Time: 5 Minutes

Cook Time: 1hr 15 Minutes

Servings: 8

Ingredients

For the Brine:

- 4 cups Water
- ¼ cup Table Salt
- ½ cup Pure Maple Syrup
- 4 cloves Garlic crushed
- 1 tablespoon Black Pepper
- 2 tablespoons Dried Rosemary

For the Roast:

- 3½ pounds Boneless Pork Loin Roast
- 1 tablespoon Canola Oil
- ⅛ teaspoon Kosher Salt
- ⅙ teaspoon Black Pepper
- For the Mustard Crust and Glaze:
- ⅓ cup Pure Maple Syrup
- 3 tablespoons Dijon Mustard
- 2 tablespoons Plain Bread Crumbs
- 1 tablespoon Buttery Spread melted

Instructions

Brine the Roast:

1. You need a container with a lid that is large enough to fit the pork loin roast.
2. Pour water into container. Add salt, maple syrup, garlic, pepper. and rosemary. Whisk together until salt is dissolved. Add the pork loin roast. Pork should be fully submerged. Place a small plate on top if needed. Cover and refrigerate overnight.

Roast the Pork:

1. Preheat oven to 450°F. Remove the pork from the brine and pat dry with paper towels.
2. Rub the roast with oil and season with salt and pepper. Place the roast fatter side down in small roasting pan. Roast in preheated oven for 15 minutes.
3. While the pork is roasting, make the mustard crust and glaze. In a small bowl, mix the maple syrup and mustard. In another small bowl, mix the melted butter with the bread crumbs.
4. Remove pork from oven and reduce temperature to 325°F. Turn the pork over so fat side is facing up. Spread the maple mustard mixture generously over top of pork. Remaining mixture can be used for serving. Sprinkle the buttery bread crumbs on top.
5. Return pork to oven and roast for another 45-60 minutes, or until the internal temperature reaches 155°F. Remove from oven and let pork rest for at least 15 minutes.
6. Maple Brined Roast Pork Loin with Mustard Glaze after cooking.

Plate and Serve:

1. Slice roast into 8 servings. Drizzle remaining maple mustard mixture over meat slices and serve.

29. Chicken Alfredo Stuffed Shells

Prep Time: 20 Minutes

Cook Time: 40 Minutes

Servings: 8

Ingredients

- 24 whole Jumbo Pasta Shells
- 1 cup Cooked Chicken such as Salt Free Baked Chicken Master Mix
- ½ cup Part Skim Ricotta Cheese
- ½ cup Low Fat Cottage Cheese
- 2 ounces Part Skim Mozzarella Cheese fine shred
- 4 ounces Parmesan Cheese grated
- 2 large Eggs
- ¼ cup Fresh Parsley chopped
- ¼ teaspoon Kosher Salt
- ¼ teaspoon Black Pepper
- 2 tablespoons Fresh Basil minced
- 4 tablespoons Buttery Spread
- 2 tablespoon All Purpose Flour
- 2 cups 2% Milk
- 1 cup Half and Half
- 3 cloves Garlic minced

Instructions

2. Preheat oven to 375°F. Lightly coat a 13 x 9-inch baking dish with cooking spray.

3. Cook pasta shells al dente. Drain. Place shells in a single layer on a baking sheet. This will make them not stick together and easier to fill.

Chicken and Cheese Mixture:

1. Make sure chicken is chopped or shredded small enough to fit in pasta shell.
2. In a medium bowl, combine ricotta, cottage cheese, 1 cup parmesan, eggs, 2 tablespoons parsley, salt, pepper, and chicken. Stir in 1-2 tablespoons half and half if mixture is too thick. Set aside.

Make the Sauce:

1. In a large skillet over medium heat, melt buttery spread. Sprinkle the flour over melted butter. Cook and whisk 1-2 minutes, or until the roux turns golden brown. Slowly pour in milk and half and half, whisking constantly. Cook until thickened, about 5 minutes. Remove from heat. Stir in garlic, remaining 1 cup parmesan, 1 tablespoon parsley, and the minced basil. Set aside.

Assemble the Dish:

2. Add 1 cup of sauce to bottom of baking dish. Using a spoon, fill each of the jumbo shells with a generous amount of the Chicken and Cheese mixture. Lay each filled shell face down in baking dish. Pour sauce all over the top of shells. Sprinkle with mozzarella. Bake in preheated oven for 25 minutes, or until sauce is bubbly and cheese is golden brown.

Plate and Serve:

3. 1 serving = 3 stuffed shells and a tablespoon of sauce.

30. Asian Sesame Chicken
Prep Time: 20 Minutes

Cook Time: 40 Minutes

Servings: 8

Ingredients

- ⅓ cup Avocado Oil
- ⅓ cup Unseasoned Rice Vinegar
- ¼ cup Reduced Sodium Soy Sauce
- 3 tablespoons Honey
- 1 teaspoon Toasted Sesame Oil
- ¼ teaspoon Black Pepper
- 2 pounds Boneless Skinless Chicken Breasts
- Sesame Seeds garnish

Instructions

Marinate the Chicken:

4. Tenderize the chicken with a meat tenderizer with metal blades. Place chicken in a gallon-sized freezer bag.
5. In a 2 cup glass measuring cup, stir together avocado oil, vinegar, soy sauce, honey, sesame oil, and pepper. Pour marinade into freezer bag with chicken. Seal bag. Place the bag in fridge (lay flat) overnight. Flip at least once.

Bake the Chicken:

1. Preheat oven to 400°F. Line a baking sheet with foil.

2. Remove chicken from marinade and place on prepared baking sheet. Discard Marinade. Bake in preheated oven for 20-25 minutes or until firm to the touch. Remove from oven and let rest for 10 minutes.

Plate and Serve:

1. Slice chicken and divide evenly between six plates. Garnish with sesame seeds.

Freeze for Later:

2. Marinate the chicken as directed. Place freezer bag in freezer for up to 5 months. When ready to cook, thaw in refrigerator and cook as directed above.